OSTEOPOROSIS DIET COOKBOOK FOR SENIORS

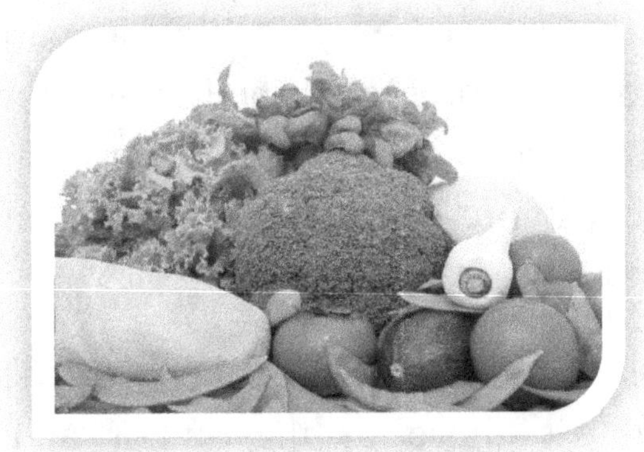

The Ultimate Nutrition Guide with Calcium rich and nutrient-dense Recipes for Bone health

Dr. Mary D. Cook

DEDICATION

To my dearest grandmother,

In the pages of this cookbook, your spirit resides—a testament to resilience, strength, and the enduring power of love. It was your journey, your whispers of pain that ignited the spark within me to delve into the healing wonders of nutrition. As I extend this guide to others, it is with gratitude and an overflow of love, for you were my inspiration and the beating heart behind every recipe. This book is dedicated to you, a celebration of your spirit, your fortitude, and the legacy of wellness you've bestowed upon our family.

With love,

{Dr. Mary D. Cook}

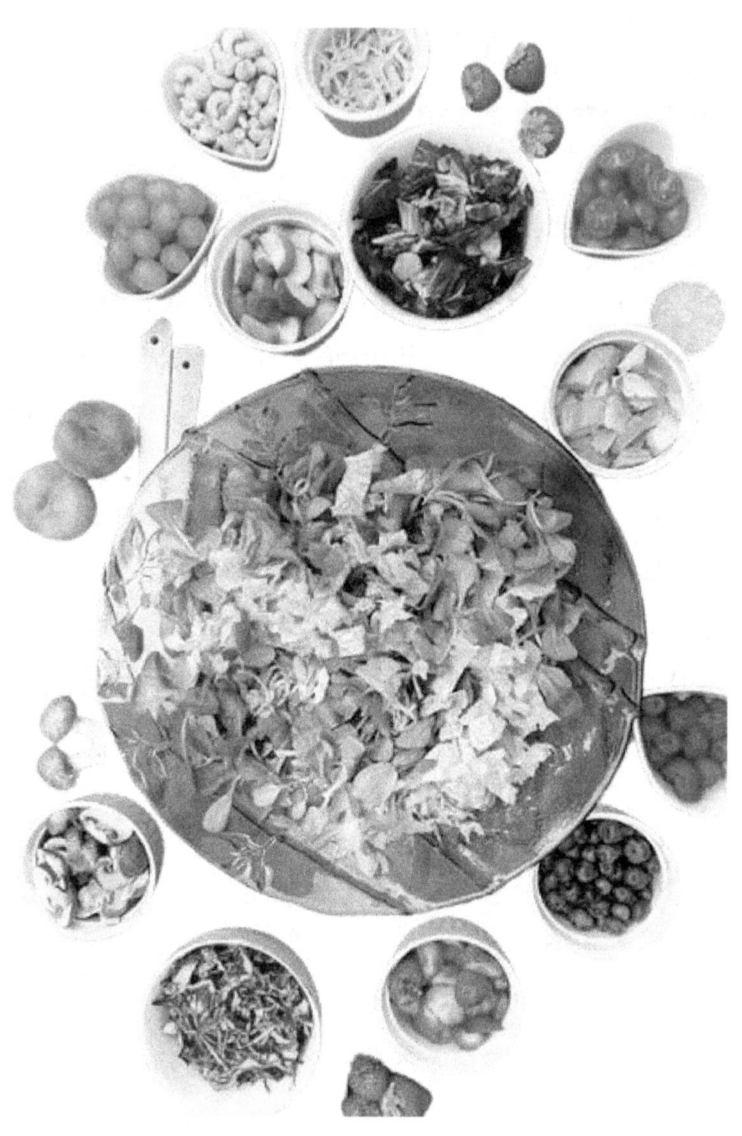

TABLE OF CONTENTS

INTRODUCTION

Greetings, dear reader,

Welcome to a culinary journey that transcends the ordinary, a journey designed not just to tantalize your taste buds but to fortify the very foundation of your vitality. I am **Dr. Mary D. Cook**, a passionate nutritionist with years of dedicated exploration into the realms of health and well-being. As your guide through the pages of this cookbook, I invite you to embark on a delicious odyssey tailored especially for seniors navigating the nuances of bone health.

In the tapestry of life, our bones are the steadfast threads that weave our stories. They deserve not just attention but a symphony of flavors that nourish them from within. The **"Osteoporosis Diet Cookbook for Seniors"** is more than a compendium of recipes; it is a manifesto for embracing the power of nutrition in the quest for resilient bones and a vibrant life.

Allow me to share a tale close to my heart, a narrative that encapsulates the very essence of why I, Dr. Mary D. Cook, am driven to guide you on this gastronomic odyssey toward better bone health.

In the quiet corners of my memories, there exists a story of resilience embodied by my beloved grandmother. Time had etched its marks on her, not just in the lines on her face but in the whispers of pain that emanated from her bones. Osteoporosis, a silent predator, had stealthily crept into her life, casting shadows of discomfort and fragility.

Witnessing her navigate the labyrinth of daily life with aching bones became my catalyst for delving deeper into the profound connection between nutrition and well-being. Armed with my passion for nutrition and an unwavering love for my grandmother, I embarked on a mission—a mission to alleviate her pain, restore her vitality, and infuse joy back into her life.

The journey was not without its challenges, but every setback fueled my determination to uncover the transformative power of food. Guided by my knowledge as a nutritionist, I curated a specialized diet that not only appeased her palate but also served as a balm for her bones. The alchemy of nutrient-dense recipes, carefully chosen ingredients, and the warmth of a granddaughter's love began to weave a tapestry of healing.

As the seasons unfolded, so did the metamorphosis within her. The twinkle returned to her eyes, and the grace with which she moved transcended the limitations that osteoporosis had imposed. The recipes that had once been mere concoctions in my kitchen became the elixir of her newfound vigor. Witnessing this transformation was a testament to the profound impact that the right nutrition can have on one's life.

Picture this cookbook as a trusted friend, a companion on your journey to stronger bones and better well-being. Within these pages, we'll unravel the mysteries of osteoporosis,

Explore the nuances of risk factors, and celebrate the prowess of ingredients that nature has bestowed upon us. From calcium-rich wonders to nutrient-dense creations, each recipe is a culinary masterpiece that fuses the science of nutrition with the art of savoring life.

So, join me in this culinary adventure—a voyage where each bite is a step towards a healthier you. Together, let's infuse joy into cooking, embrace the vibrancy of flavors, and cultivate a lifestyle that not only satiates the palate but fortifies the very essence of your being. Your journey to resilient bones and a more vibrant you begins here—where every recipe is crafted with love, knowledge, and the unwavering belief that good food is the cornerstone of a flourishing life.

Bon appétit, and here's to a future where each meal is a celebration of your enduring vitality.

Warm regards,

{Dr. Mary D. Cook}

CHAPTER 1:
Understanding Osteoporosis

1.1 What is Osteoporosis?

Osteoporosis is a medical condition characterized by the weakening of bones, making them fragile and more susceptible to fractures. It occurs when the density and quality of bone are reduced, leading to a porous and brittle structure. The word "osteoporosis" literally means "porous bone."

In a healthy bone, there is a continuous process of bone tissue breakdown and rebuilding. However, in individuals with osteoporosis, the creation of new bone doesn't keep up with the removal of old bone. This imbalance results in bones becoming porous, weak, and prone to fractures, even with minor stress or falls.

Osteoporosis often progresses without noticeable symptoms until a fracture occurs, typically in the hip, spine, or wrist. It is more common in older adults, especially postmenopausal women, as hormonal changes during menopause can contribute to bone loss. Additionally, certain medical conditions and medications can increase the risk of developing osteoporosis.

Preventive measures include a diet rich in calcium and vitamin D, regular weight-bearing exercises, and lifestyle modifications. Early detection through bone density testing and appropriate medical intervention can help manage and treat osteoporosis effectively.

1.2 The Impact on Senior Health

Osteoporosis can have significant impacts on senior health, affecting various aspects of well-being. Here are some key areas where osteoporosis can have an impact:

1. **Increased Risk of Fractures:** Osteoporosis weakens bones, making them more susceptible to fractures. Seniors with osteoporosis are at a higher risk of experiencing fractures, especially in the hip, spine, and wrist. These fractures can lead to pain, loss of mobility, and a decline in overall quality of life.

2. **Pain and Discomfort:** Fractures and bone loss associated with osteoporosis can result in chronic pain and discomfort. This can affect daily activities, mobility, and independence, leading to a reduced quality of life for seniors.

3. **Changes in Posture and Height Loss:** Osteoporosis can cause the vertebrae in the spine to weaken and collapse, leading to changes in posture and height loss. This can contribute to a stooped or hunched appearance, impacting both physical and psychological well-being.

4. **Decreased Muscle Strength:** As a consequence of fractures and reduced physical activity due to pain, muscle strength may decline.

Weakened muscles can further contribute to mobility issues and an increased risk of falls.

4. Diminished Quality of Life: The combination of fractures, pain, changes in posture, and reduced mobility can collectively diminish the overall quality of life for seniors with osteoporosis. The condition may limit their ability to engage in social activities, hobbies, and daily tasks.

5. Increased Healthcare Costs: Osteoporosis-related fractures often require medical attention, hospitalization, and rehabilitation. The associated healthcare costs can be substantial, both for individuals and the healthcare system.

6. Emotional Impact: Dealing with the physical consequences of osteoporosis, such as pain, fractures, and changes in appearance, can have emotional repercussions. Seniors may experience anxiety, depression, or a decreased sense of well-being.

Understanding these impacts emphasizes the importance of proactive measures, such as preventive lifestyle choices, proper nutrition, and medical management, to maintain bone health and reduce the risk and consequences of osteoporosis in seniors.

1.3 Identifying Risk Factors

Identifying the risk factors for osteoporosis is crucial for early detection and effective prevention. Several factors contribute to an increased risk of developing osteoporosis, and understanding these can help individuals take proactive measures to maintain bone health. Here are some key risk factors:

1. Age: The risk of osteoporosis increases with age, particularly in postmenopausal women. The aging process can lead to a decrease in bone density and an increased likelihood of fractures.

2. Gender: Women, especially postmenopausal women, are at a higher risk of developing osteoporosis. The decline in estrogen levels during menopause contributes to bone loss.

3. Family History: A family history of osteoporosis or fractures may increase an individual's risk. Genetics can play a role in determining bone density and susceptibility to fractures.

4. Body Weight and Composition: Low body weight and a small, slender frame can be risk factors for osteoporosis. Individuals with less bone mass to start with may be at a higher risk.

5. Hormonal Changes: Hormonal imbalances, such as low estrogen levels in women and low testosterone levels in men, can contribute to bone loss.

6. Nutritional Deficiencies: Inadequate intake of calcium and vitamin D, essential nutrients for bone health, can increase the risk of osteoporosis. Poor nutrition, especially in the formative years, may have long-term consequences for bone density.

7. Lifestyle Factors: Certain lifestyle choices can contribute to osteoporosis. These include smoking, excessive alcohol consumption, and a sedentary lifestyle.

Smoking interferes with the absorption of calcium, while excessive alcohol can negatively impact bone formation.

8. Medical Conditions and Medications: Some medical conditions, such as rheumatoid arthritis, celiac disease, and hormonal disorders, can affect bone health. Additionally, long-term use of certain medications, like corticosteroids, can contribute to bone loss.

9. Lack of Physical Activity: Insufficient weight-bearing exercise, which includes activities like walking, jogging, and resistance training, can lead to decreased bone density.

10. Previous Fractures: Individuals who have experienced fractures in the past may be at an increased risk of developing osteoporosis, as fractures can indicate compromised bone strength.

Identifying these risk factors allows individuals and healthcare professionals to assess the likelihood of osteoporosis and take preventive measures.

Lifestyle modifications, proper nutrition, weight-bearing exercises, and regular bone density screenings can help manage and reduce the risk of osteoporosis.

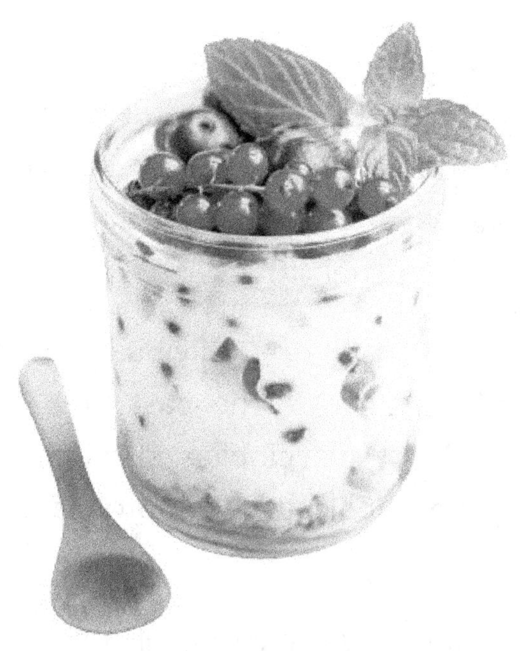

CHAPTER 2:
Building Strong Bones Through Nutrition

2.1 The Role of Calcium in Bone Health

Calcium plays a crucial role in maintaining and promoting optimal bone health throughout the lifespan. Here are the key roles of calcium in supporting bone health:

1. Bone Structure and Density: Calcium is a primary component of bone tissue, providing the structural framework that gives bones their strength and density. Adequate calcium intake is essential for the formation of a strong and resilient skeletal system.

2. Bone Formation: During periods of bone growth, such as childhood, adolescence, and early adulthood, calcium is instrumental in the process of bone formation.

It helps in the development of a dense and healthy bone structure, laying the foundation for lifelong skeletal integrity.

3. Bone Remodeling: Bone is a dynamic tissue that undergoes constant remodeling, involving the removal of old bone and the formation of new bone. Calcium, along with other minerals, is actively involved in this remodeling process, ensuring that bones remain strong and resilient.

4. Blood Clotting: Calcium plays a critical role in blood clotting, contributing to the formation of a stable blood clot when there is an injury. This function is vital for preventing excessive bleeding in the event of injuries or wounds.

5. Muscle Contraction: Calcium is essential for muscle contraction, including the contraction of skeletal muscles that move the body. When muscles contract, calcium ions are released, facilitating the interaction between proteins that generates force and movement.

6. **Nerve Function:** Calcium is involved in transmitting signals between nerve cells and facilitating the release of neurotransmitters. Proper nerve function is crucial for various physiological processes, including the coordination of muscle movements and the maintenance of overall body balance.

7. **Cell Signaling:** Calcium serves as a secondary messenger in various cellular signaling pathways. It plays a role in regulating a wide range of cellular activities, contributing to the overall health and function of different cell types in the body.

8. **Hormone Secretion:** Calcium is involved in the release of hormones, including those that regulate bone metabolism. Parathyroid hormone (PTH) and calcitonin, for example, are hormones that help regulate calcium levels in the blood and influence bone turnover.

To maintain optimal bone health, it's essential to obtain an adequate amount of calcium through dietary sources such as dairy products, leafy green vegetables, fortified foods, and supplements when necessary.

Ensuring sufficient calcium intake is especially important during periods of rapid growth, such as childhood and adolescence, and in later years to prevent age-related bone loss and conditions like osteoporosis.

2.2 Essential Vitamins and Minerals for Bone Strength

Several essential vitamins and minerals play a crucial role in maintaining bone strength and promoting overall bone health. Here are key nutrients that contribute to bone strength:

1. Calcium: As previously mentioned, calcium is a primary mineral that forms the structural basis of bones and teeth. It is vital for bone density, strength, and the prevention of osteoporosis.

2. Vitamin D: Vitamin D is essential for the absorption of calcium in the intestines. It helps regulate calcium and phosphorus levels in the blood and supports the formation and mineralization of bone.

Exposure to sunlight is a natural way to synthesize vitamin D, and it is also found in some foods and supplements.

3. Vitamin K: Vitamin K is involved in the synthesis of proteins that regulate bone mineralization. It helps in binding calcium to the bone matrix, contributing to bone strength. Leafy green vegetables, such as kale and spinach, are good sources of vitamin K.

4. Magnesium: Magnesium is a mineral that works in conjunction with calcium to support bone health. It is involved in bone mineralization and the activation of vitamin D. Nuts, seeds, whole grains, and leafy green vegetables are good sources of magnesium.

5. Phosphorus: Phosphorus is another mineral that forms a major component of bone mineralization. It works in tandem with calcium to provide strength and structure to bones. Dairy products, meat, fish, and whole grains are common sources of phosphorus.

6. **Vitamin C:** Vitamin C is essential for collagen synthesis, which is a key component of the bone matrix. Collagen provides a framework for the mineralization of bone. Citrus fruits, berries, and vegetables like broccoli are good sources of vitamin C.

7. **Vitamin A:** Vitamin A is involved in bone remodeling and the maintenance of bone density. It supports the differentiation of bone cells and helps regulate bone turnover. Foods rich in vitamin A include sweet potatoes, carrots, and leafy green vegetables.

8. **Zinc:** Zinc is a trace element that plays a role in bone mineralization and the synthesis of collagen. It is involved in the formation and function of bone cells. Meat, dairy products, nuts, and seeds are good sources of zinc.

9. **Boron:** Boron is a trace mineral that may contribute to bone health by influencing calcium and magnesium metabolism. It is found in fruits, vegetables, and nuts.

10. Vitamin E: Vitamin E is an antioxidant that may help protect bones from oxidative stress. Nuts, seeds, and vegetable oils are good sources of vitamin E.

A balanced and varied diet that includes a mix of these vitamins and minerals, along with regular physical activity, contributes to maintaining optimal bone health throughout life. It's important to note that these nutrients work synergistically, and a deficiency in one may impact the effectiveness of others. As always, individual dietary needs can vary, and consulting with a healthcare professional or registered dietitian is advisable for personalized guidance.

2.3 Incorporating Plant-Based Nutrients

Incorporating plant-based nutrients into your diet is a wonderful way to support bone health while embracing the benefits of a plant-centric lifestyle. Here are key plant-based nutrients and ways to include them in your diet for optimal bone health:

1. Leafy Green Vegetables:

Nutrients: Rich in calcium, magnesium, vitamin K, and various antioxidants.

Incorporation: Include spinach, kale, collard greens, and bok choy in salads, smoothies, stir-fries, or as side dishes.

2. Tofu and Tempeh:

Nutrients: Excellent sources of calcium and protein.

Incorporation: Use tofu and tempeh in stir-fries, salads, soups, or marinate and grill for a delicious main dish.

3. Legumes (Beans and Lentils):

Nutrients: Provide calcium, magnesium, phosphorus, and protein.

Incorporation: Include beans and lentils in soups, stews, salads, or as a meat substitute in various dishes.

Nutrients: Contain calcium, magnesium, phosphorus, and healthy fats.

Incorporation: Snack on almonds, sesame seeds, chia seeds, or add them to cereals, yogurt, salads, or smoothies.

Nutrients: Supply magnesium, phosphorus, and various B vitamins.

Incorporation: Choose whole grains like quinoa, brown rice, oats, and whole wheat bread for a nutrient-dense base in meals.

Nutrients: Fortified with calcium, vitamin D, and vitamin B12.

Incorporation: Use fortified almond, soy, or oat milk in cereals, coffee, and cooking as a dairy alternative.

7. Fortified Foods:

Nutrients: Look for plant-based foods fortified with calcium and vitamin D.

Incorporation: Incorporate fortified tofu, cereals, and nutritional yeast into your meals for an extra nutrient boost.

8. Colorful Fruits:

Nutrients: Provide vitamin C, antioxidants, and other beneficial compounds.

Incorporation: Enjoy a variety of fruits such as oranges, berries, kiwi, and mangoes as snacks or in fruit salads.

9. Seaweed:

Nutrients: Rich in calcium, magnesium, and trace minerals.

Incorporation: Include seaweed in soups, salads, or as a wrap for sushi rolls to enhance mineral intake.

Nutrients: Some herbs and spices contain bone-supporting nutrients.

Incorporation: Use herbs like parsley, thyme, and spices like turmeric in cooking for added flavor and nutrients.

Remember to focus on a well-balanced diet that includes a variety of plant-based foods to ensure you receive a broad spectrum of nutrients that contribute to overall bone health. If needed, consider consulting with a nutritionist or dietitian for personalized advice tailored to your specific dietary preferences and health goals.

2.4 Stocking Your Pantry for Osteoporosis Support

Stocking your pantry with nutrient-rich foods is a proactive step in supporting bone health and managing osteoporosis. Here's a guide to stocking a bone-friendly pantry:

1. Whole Grains:

Quinoa, brown rice, oats, whole wheat pasta, and whole grain bread provide magnesium, phosphorus, and B vitamins.

2. Legumes:

Stock up on beans (black beans, chickpeas, lentils) for a plant-based protein source that also offers calcium and magnesium.

3. Nuts and Seeds:

Almonds, walnuts, chia seeds, and flaxseeds are rich in calcium, magnesium, and healthy fats.

4. Fortified Foods:

Choose fortified tofu, plant-based milk (almond, soy, oat), and breakfast cereals to ensure an adequate intake of calcium and vitamin D.

5. Leafy Greens:

Keep spinach, kale, collard greens, and Swiss chard for their high calcium, vitamin K, and magnesium content.

6. Canned Fish with Bones:

Opt for canned salmon or sardines, which provide both calcium and vitamin D from the bones.

7. Seaweed:

Include dried seaweed or nori sheets in your pantry for their calcium and magnesium content.

8. Herbs and Spices:

Garlic, turmeric, thyme, and parsley not only add flavor but also offer bone-supporting nutrients.

9. Whole Fruits:

Have a variety of fruits, especially those rich in vitamin C (oranges, berries, kiwi) for collagen formation.

10. Dried Fruits:

Prunes and dried figs are good sources of calcium and can be a tasty addition to snacks or desserts.

11. Canned Tomatoes:

Tomatoes are rich in vitamin C and lycopene, which may support bone health.

12. Olive Oil:

Use extra virgin olive oil for cooking; it contains healthy fats and antioxidants.

13. Canned or Dried Beans:

A convenient source of plant-based protein, fiber, and essential minerals.

14. Whole-Grain Snacks:

Keep whole-grain crackers, rice cakes, or air-popped popcorn for nutritious snack options.

15. Low-Sodium Broth:

Vegetable or bone broth can be a base for soups, providing additional nutrients.

16. Non-Dairy Yogurt:

Choose fortified plant-based yogurts for calcium and vitamin D.

17. Herbal Teas:

Chamomile and nettle teas are caffeine-free options that may have bone-supporting properties.

18. Dark Chocolate:

In moderation, dark chocolate can contribute magnesium and other minerals.

Remember to check food labels for nutritional information, especially regarding calcium and vitamin D content. Additionally, aim for a well-balanced diet with a variety of foods to ensure you're getting a broad spectrum of nutrients essential for bone health. Regularly reassess and replenish your pantry to maintain a consistent supply of bone-friendly foods.

7-DAY MEAL PLAN

DAY-1:

Breakfast: Spinach and Feta Omelette {Pg. 39}

Lunch: Turkey and Vegetable Stir-Fry {Pg. 55}

Dinner: Shrimp and Zucchini Noodles Stir-Fry {Pg 71 }

Snack: Apple and Walnut Salad {Pg. 87}

DAY-2:

Breakfast: Veggie Breakfast Burrito {Pg. 46}

Lunch: Greek Chickpea Salad {Pg. 54}

Dinner: Salmon and Asparagus Foil Packets {Pg. 67}

Snack: Cucumber and Hummus Rolls {Pg. 92}

DAY-3:

Breakfast: Calcium-Rich Breakfast Smoothie {Pg.37}

Lunch: Salmon and Quinoa Salad **{Pg.52}**

Dinner: Cabbage and Lentil Soup **{Pg. 72}**

Snack: Peach and Mint Salsa **{Pg.94}**

DAY-4:

Breakfast: Oatmeal with Almond Milk and Berries **{Pg. 42}**

Lunch: Egg Salad Lettuce Wraps **{Pg. 57}**

Dinner: Quinoa and Broccoli Bowl with Tofu **{Pg.77}**

Snack: Cherry Almond Frozen Yogurt Popsicles **{Pg.95}**

DAY-5:

Breakfast: Avocado and Tomato Breakfast Toast **{Pg.38}**

Lunch: Mushroom and Spinach Stuffed Chicken **{Pg.53} Breast**

Dinner: Turkey and Sweet Potato Skillet **{Pg. 76}**

Snack: Coconut Yogurt and Mango Parfait **{Pg. 89}**

DAY-6:

Breakfast: Smoked Salmon and Cream Cheese Bagel **{Pg. 43}**

Lunch: Quinoa and Black Bean Bowl **{Pg.56}**

Dinner: Lentil and Vegetable Stuffed Peppers **{Pg.73}**

Snack: Cherry Almond Frozen Yogurt Popsicles **{Pg.95}**

DAY-7:

Breakfast: Chia Seed Pudding **{Pg.40}**

Lunch: Cabbage and Apple Slaw with Grilled Chicken **{Pg.64}**

Dinner: Cauliflower and Broccoli Soup **{Pg. 62}**

Snack: Mango Sorbet **{Pg.91}**

CHAPTER 3:
Calcium-Rich Recipes for Everyday Wellness

Breakfast Boosters: Start Your Day with Bone-Nourishing Meals

1. Calcium-Rich Breakfast Smoothie

Ingredients:

- 1 cup fortified almond milk
- 1/2 cup Greek yogurt
- 1/2 cup fresh spinach
- 1/2 banana
- 1 tablespoon chia seeds

Instructions:

1. Blend all ingredients until smooth.
2. Pour into a glass and enjoy!

Servings: 1   **Cooking Time:** 5 minutes

Nutritional Value: Calories: 250, Calcium: 400 mg, Vitamin D: 120 IU

2. Avocado and Tomato Breakfast Toast

Ingredients:

- 1 slice whole-grain bread
- 1/2 avocado, mashed
- 1 small tomato, sliced
- Sprinkle of sesame seeds
- Salt and pepper to taste

Instructions:

1. Toast the bread to your liking.
2. Spread mashed avocado on the toast.
3. Arrange tomato slices on top.
4. Sprinkle with sesame seeds, salt, and pepper.

Servings: 1

Nutritional Value:

- Calories: 280
- Calcium: 120 mg
- Vitamin D: 80 IU

Cooking Time: 7 minutes

3. Spinach and Feta Omelette

Ingredients:

- 2 eggs
- Handful of fresh spinach
- 2 tablespoons crumbled feta cheese
- Salt and pepper to taste

Instructions:

1. Whisk eggs in a bowl.
2. Sauté spinach in a pan until wilted.
3. Pour eggs over the spinach, add feta, and cook until set.
4. Season with salt and pepper.

Servings: 1

Nutritional Value:

- Calories: 320
- Calcium: 200 mg
- Vitamin D: 60 IU

Cooking Time: 10 minutes

4. Chia Seed Pudding

Ingredients:

- 2 tablespoons chia seeds
- 1 cup fortified coconut milk
- 1/2 teaspoon vanilla extract
- Fresh berries for topping

Instructions:

1. Mix chia seeds, coconut milk, and vanilla in a bowl.
2. Refrigerate overnight or for at least 2 hours.
3. Top with fresh berries before serving.

Servings: 1

Nutritional Value:

- Calories: 180
- Calcium: 220 mg
- Vitamin D: 100 IU

Preparation Time: 5 minutes (plus chilling time)

5. Greek Yogurt Parfait

Ingredients:

- 1 cup Greek yogurt
- 1/4 cup granola
- Handful of sliced strawberries
- Drizzle of honey

Instructions:

1. Layer Greek yogurt, granola, and strawberries in a glass.
2. Drizzle with honey before serving.

Servings: 1

Nutritional Value:

- Calories: 280
- Calcium: 300 mg
- Vitamin D: 80 IU

Assembly Time: 5 minutes

Ingredients:

- 1/2 cup rolled oats
- 1 cup fortified almond milk
- Handful of mixed berries
- 1 tablespoon chopped almonds

Instructions:

1. Cook oats in almond milk according to package instructions.
2. Top with mixed berries and chopped almonds.

Servings: 1

Nutritional Value:

- Calories: 270
- Calcium: 250 mg
- Vitamin D: 120 IU

Cooking Time: 5 minutes

7. Smoked Salmon and Cream Cheese Bagel

Ingredients:

- 1 whole-grain bagel
- 2 tablespoons low-fat cream cheese
- 2 slices smoked salmon
- Sliced cucumber and capers for topping

Instructions:

1. Toast the bagel to your liking.
2. Spread cream cheese on each half.
3. Top with smoked salmon, cucumber, and capers.

Servings: 1

Nutritional Value:

- Calories: 340
- Calcium: 200 mg
- Vitamin D: 90 IU

Assembly Time: 7 minutes

8. Blueberry and Almond Pancakes

Ingredients:

- 1/2 cup whole wheat pancake mix
- 1/2 cup fortified soy milk
- Handful of fresh blueberries
- 1 tablespoon chopped almonds

Instructions:

1. Mix pancake mix and soy milk until smooth.
2. Fold in blueberries.
3. Cook pancakes on a griddle and sprinkle with chopped almonds.

Servings: 1

Nutritional Value:

- Calories: 320
- Calcium: 180 mg
- Vitamin D: 80 IU

Cooking Time: 10 minutes

9. Cottage Cheese and Pineapple Bowl

Ingredients:

- 1/2 cup low-fat cottage cheese
- 1/2 cup fresh pineapple chunks
- 1 tablespoon sunflower seeds

Instructions:

1. Combine cottage cheese and pineapple in a bowl.
2. Sprinkle with sunflower seeds.

Servings: 1

Nutritional Value:

- Calories: 220
- Calcium: 150 mg
- Vitamin D: 70 IU

Assembly Time: 5 minutes

10. Veggie Breakfast Burrito

Ingredients:

- 1 whole wheat tortilla
- 2 eggs, scrambled
- Salsa
- Sliced avocado
- Chopped cilantro

Instructions:

1. Fill tortilla with scrambled eggs.
2. Top with salsa, sliced avocado, and cilantro.
3. Roll into a burrito.

Servings: 1

Nutritional Value:

- Calories: 320
- Calcium: 170 mg
- Vitamin D: 60 IU

Cooking Time: 8 minutes

11. Almond Butter and Banana Wrap

Ingredients:

- 1 whole grain wrap
- 2 tablespoons almond butter
- 1 banana, sliced
- Drizzle of honey

Instructions:

1. Spread almond butter on the wrap.
2. Add sliced banana and drizzle with honey.
3. Roll into a wrap.

Servings: 1

Nutritional Value:

- Calories: 290
- Calcium: 120 mg
- Vitamin D: 80 IU

Assembly Time: 5 minutes

12. Mango and Coconut Chia Pudding

Ingredients:

- 2 tablespoons chia seeds
- 1 cup fortified coconut milk
- 1/2 cup diced mango

Instructions:

1. Mix chia seeds and coconut milk in a bowl.
2. Refrigerate until set.
3. Top with diced mango before serving.

Servings: 1

Nutritional Value:

- Calories: 260
- Calcium: 210 mg
- Vitamin D: 90 IU

Preparation Time: 5 minutes (plus chilling time)

Ingredients:

- 1 small sweet potato, grated
- Handful of kale, chopped
- 1 egg
- 1 tablespoon olive oil

Instructions:

1. Sauté grated sweet potato and kale in olive oil until cooked.
2. Fry an egg and place on top of the hash.

Servings: 1

Nutritional Value:

- Calories: 280
- Calcium: 120 mg
- Vitamin D: 70 IU

Cooking Time: 10 minutes

14. Pumpkin Pie Overnight Oats

Ingredients:

- 1/2 cup rolled oats
- 1/2 cup fortified pumpkin puree
- 1/2 teaspoon pumpkin spice
- 1 tablespoon maple syrup

Instructions:

1. Mix oats, pumpkin puree, pumpkin spice, and maple syrup.
2. Refrigerate overnight.
3. Enjoy cold or heat in the morning.

Servings: 1

Nutritional Value:

- Calories: 290
- Calcium: 150 mg
- Vitamin D: 80 IU

Preparation Time: 5 minutes (plus chilling time)

15. Cherry Almond Protein Smoothie

Ingredients:

- 1 cup fortified almond milk
- 1/2 cup frozen cherries
- 1 scoop plant-based protein powder
- 1 tablespoon almond butter

Instructions:

1. Blend almond milk, frozen cherries, protein powder, and almond butter until smooth.
2. Pour into a glass and enjoy!

Servings: 1

Nutritional Value:

- Calories: 300
- Calcium: 200 mg
- Vitamin D: 120 IU

Cooking Time: 5 minutes

Lunchtime Favorites: Delicious Midday Recipes for Strong Bones

1. Salmon and Quinoa Salad

Ingredients:

- 4 oz grilled salmon
- 1/2 cup cooked quinoa
- Mixed salad greens
- Cherry tomatoes, sliced
- 1 tablespoon olive oil
- Lemon juice, salt, and pepper to taste

Instructions:

1. Combine grilled salmon, quinoa, salad greens, and tomatoes in a bowl.
2. Drizzle with olive oil and lemon juice.
3. Season with salt and pepper.

Servings: 1

Nutritional Value: Calories: 400, Calcium: 200 mg, Vitamin D: 300 IU

Cooking Time: 15 minutes

2. Mushroom and Spinach Stuffed Chicken Breast

Ingredients:

- 1 boneless, skinless chicken breast
- 1/2 cup sautéed mushrooms and spinach
- 1 teaspoon olive oil
- Garlic powder, salt, and pepper to taste

Instructions:

1. Cut a pocket into the chicken breast.
2. Stuff with sautéed mushrooms and spinach.
3. Season with garlic powder, salt, and pepper.
4. Bake until chicken is cooked through.

Servings: 1

Nutritional Value:

- Calories: 350
- Calcium: 180 mg
- Vitamin D: 120 IU

Cooking Time: 25 minutes

Ingredients:

- 1 cup canned chickpeas, rinsed
- Cucumber, diced
- Cherry tomatoes, halved
- Red onion, finely chopped
- Feta cheese, crumbled
- Olive oil, balsamic vinegar, oregano, salt, and pepper to taste

Instructions:

1. Combine chickpeas, cucumber, tomatoes, red onion, and feta in a bowl.
2. Drizzle with olive oil and balsamic vinegar.
3. Season with oregano, salt, and pepper.

Servings: 1

Nutritional Value:

- Calories: 380
- Calcium: 180 mg
- Vitamin D: 90 IU

Preparation Time: 10 minutes

4. Turkey and Vegetable Stir-Fry

Ingredients:

- 4 oz ground turkey
- Mixed stir-fry vegetables (broccoli, bell peppers, snap peas)
- 1 tablespoon low-sodium soy sauce
- 1 teaspoon sesame oil
- Ginger and garlic, minced
- Brown rice, cooked

Instructions:

1. Cook ground turkey in a pan until browned.
2. Add mixed vegetables, soy sauce, sesame oil, ginger, and garlic.
3. Stir-fry until vegetables are tender.
4. Serve over cooked brown rice.

Servings: 1

Nutritional Value: Calories: 420, Calcium: 120 mg

Vitamin D: 80 IU

Cooking Time: 20 minutes

5. Quinoa and Black Bean Bowl

Ingredients:

- 1/2 cup cooked quinoa
- 1/2 cup canned black beans, rinsed
- Avocado, sliced
- Salsa
- Fresh cilantro, chopped
- Lime wedges

Instructions:

1. Mix quinoa and black beans in a bowl.
2. Top with sliced avocado, salsa, and cilantro.
3. Squeeze lime wedges over the bowl.

Servings: 1

Nutritional Value:

- Calories: 350
- Calcium: 180 mg
- Vitamin D: 60 IU

Assembly Time: 10 minutes

Ingredients:

- 2 boiled eggs, chopped
- Greek yogurt
- Dijon mustard
- Celery, finely chopped
- Lettuce leaves for wrapping

Instructions:

1. Mix chopped eggs, Greek yogurt, Dijon mustard, and celery.
2. Spoon onto lettuce leaves.
3. Roll into wraps.

Servings: 1

Nutritional Value:

- Calories: 280
- Calcium: 140 mg
- Vitamin D: 70 IU

Preparation Time: 15 minutes

7. Lentil and Vegetable Soup

Ingredients:

- 1/2 cup dried lentils, rinsed
- Mixed vegetables (carrots, celery, onions)
- Low-sodium vegetable broth
- Bay leaves, thyme, salt, and pepper to taste

Instructions:

1. Combine lentils, mixed vegetables, and vegetable broth in a pot.
2. Add bay leaves, thyme, salt, and pepper.
3. Simmer until lentils are tender.

Servings: 1

Nutritional Value:

- Calories: 300
- Calcium: 120 mg
- Vitamin D: 60 IU

Cooking Time: 30 minutes

8. Sweet Potato and Chickpea Buddha Bowl

Ingredients:

- Roasted sweet potato chunks
- Canned chickpeas, rinsed and roasted
- Quinoa, cooked
- Kale, massaged
- Tahini dressing

Instructions:

1. Arrange sweet potato, chickpeas, quinoa, and kale in a bowl.
2. Drizzle with tahini dressing.

Servings: 1

Nutritional Value:

- Calories: 380
- Calcium: 150 mg
- Vitamin D: 80 IU

Preparation Time: 25 minutes

9. Caprese Salad with Grilled Chicken

Ingredients:

- Grilled chicken breast
- Tomato, sliced
- Fresh mozzarella, sliced
- Fresh basil leaves
- Balsamic glaze
- Olive oil, salt, and pepper to taste

Instructions:

1. Arrange grilled chicken, tomato, and mozzarella on a plate.
2. Top with fresh basil.
3. Drizzle with balsamic glaze and olive oil.
4. Season with salt and pepper.

Servings: 1

Nutritional Value:

- Calories: 350
- Calcium: 250 mg
- Vitamin D: 120 IU

Assembly Time: 15 minutes

10. Shrimp and Asparagus Stir-Fry

Ingredients:

- Shrimp, peeled and deveined
- Asparagus, trimmed and cut into pieces
- Garlic, minced
- Low-sodium soy sauce
- Sesame oil
- Brown rice, cooked

Instructions:

1. Sauté shrimp and asparagus in sesame oil until cooked.
2. Add minced garlic and soy sauce.
3. Serve over cooked brown rice.

Servings: 1

Nutritional Value:

- Calories: 380
- Calcium: 110 mg
- Vitamin D: 80 IU

Cooking Time: 15 minutes

11. Cauliflower and Broccoli Soup

Ingredients:

- Cauliflower, chopped
- Broccoli, chopped
- Low-sodium vegetable broth
- Onion, garlic, salt, and pepper to taste

Instructions:

1. Cook cauliflower and broccoli in vegetable broth until tender.
2. Blend until smooth.
3. Sauté onions and garlic, then add to the soup.
4. Season with salt and pepper.

Servings: 1

Nutritional Value:

- Calories: 280
- Calcium: 150 mg
- Vitamin D: 60 IU

Cooking Time: 25 minutes

12. Turkey and Spinach Wrap

Ingredients:

- Whole wheat wrap
- Sliced turkey breast
- Hummus
- Baby spinach leaves
- Cherry tomatoes, sliced
- Red onion, thinly sliced

Instructions:

1. Spread hummus on the wrap.
2. Layer with turkey, spinach, tomatoes, and red onion.
3. Roll into a wrap.

Servings: 1

Nutritional Value:

- Calories: 320
- Calcium: 120 mg
- Vitamin D: 70 IU

Assembly Time: 10 minutes

13. Cabbage and Apple Slaw with Grilled Chicken

Ingredients:

- Grilled chicken strips
- Red and green cabbage, shredded
- Apple, julienned
- Greek yogurt dressing

Instructions:

1. Toss grilled chicken, cabbage, and apple in a bowl.
2. Drizzle with Greek yogurt dressing.

Servings: 1

Nutritional Value:

- Calories: 360
- Calcium: 200 mg
- Vitamin D: 120 IU

Assembly Time: 15 minutes

14. Tomato Basil Chickpea Pasta

Ingredients:

- Whole wheat pasta
- Canned chickpeas, rinsed
- Cherry tomatoes, halved
- Fresh basil leaves
- Olive oil, garlic, salt, and pepper to taste

Instructions:

1. Cook pasta according to package instructions.
2. Sauté chickpeas and cherry tomatoes in olive oil and garlic.
3. Toss with cooked pasta and fresh basil.
4. Season with salt and pepper.

Servings: 1

Nutritional Value:

- Calories: 380
- Calcium: 180 mg
- Vitamin D: 80 IU

Cooking Time: 20 minutes

15. Spinach and Walnut Stuffed Bell Peppers

Ingredients:

- Bell peppers, halved and cleaned
- Sautéed spinach and garlic
- Quinoa, cooked
- Chopped walnuts
- Feta cheese, crumbled

Instructions:

1. Mix sautéed spinach, cooked quinoa, chopped walnuts, and feta.
2. Stuff bell peppers with the mixture.
3. Bake until peppers are tender.

Servings: 1

Nutritional Value:

- Calories: 320
- Calcium: 150 mg
- Vitamin D: 70 IU

Cooking Time: 30 minutes

Dinner Delights: Nutrient-Dense Dinners to Support Your Bones

1. Salmon and Asparagus Foil Packets

Ingredients:

- 6 oz salmon fillet
- Asparagus spears
- Lemon slices
- Olive oil, garlic, salt, and pepper to taste

Instructions:

1. Place salmon on a foil sheet.
2. Arrange asparagus around the salmon.
3. Drizzle with olive oil, add minced garlic, and season with salt and pepper.
4. Seal the foil packet and bake until salmon is cooked through.

Servings: 1

Nutritional Value: Calories: 400, Calcium: 180 mg, Vitamin D: 300 IU

Cooking Time: 20 minutes

2. Vegetarian Stuffed Bell Peppers

Ingredients:

- Bell peppers, halved and cleaned
- Quinoa, cooked
- Black beans, canned and rinsed
- Corn kernels
- Salsa
- Mexican seasoning, salt, and pepper to taste

Instructions:

1. Mix cooked quinoa, black beans, corn, salsa, and seasoning in a bowl.
2. Stuff bell peppers with the mixture.
3. Bake until peppers are tender.

Servings: 1

Nutritional Value:

Calories: 350,

Calcium: 160 mg

Vitamin D: 80 IU

Cooking Time: 30 minutes

3. Lemon Herb Grilled Chicken

Ingredients:

- 1 boneless, skinless chicken breast
- Lemon juice, olive oil, garlic, rosemary, thyme, salt, and pepper to taste

Instructions:

1. Marinate chicken in lemon juice, olive oil, minced garlic, and herbs.
2. Grill until cooked through.

Servings: 1

Nutritional Value:

- Calories: 320
- Calcium: 150 mg
- Vitamin D: 100 IU

Cooking Time: 15 minutes

4. Eggplant and Tomato Bake

Ingredients:

- 1 medium eggplant, sliced
- Tomato, sliced
- Mozzarella cheese, shredded
- Fresh basil leaves
- Olive oil, garlic, salt, and pepper to taste

Instructions:

1. Layer eggplant and tomato slices in a baking dish.
2. Drizzle with olive oil, add minced garlic, and season with salt and pepper.
3. Top with shredded mozzarella.
4. Bake until cheese is melted and bubbly.

Servings: 1

Nutritional Value:

- Calories: 340
- Calcium: 200 mg
- Vitamin D: 90 IU

Cooking Time: 25 minutes

Ingredients:

- Shrimp, peeled and deveined
- Zucchini, spiralized into noodles
- Bell peppers, sliced
- Low-sodium soy sauce
- Sesame oil, garlic, ginger, salt, and pepper to taste

Instructions:

1. Sauté shrimp, zucchini noodles, and bell peppers in sesame oil.
2. Add minced garlic, ginger, soy sauce, salt, and pepper.
3. Stir-fry until shrimp are cooked.

Servings: 1

Nutritional Value:

- Calories: 280
- Calcium: 120 mg
- Vitamin D: 80 IU

Cooking Time: 15 minutes

6. Mushroom and Spinach Frittata

Ingredients:

- 2 eggs
- Mushrooms, sliced
- Fresh spinach leaves
- Onion, diced
- Feta cheese, crumbled
- Olive oil, salt, and pepper to taste

Instructions:

1. Sauté mushrooms and onions in olive oil until softened.
2. Add fresh spinach and cook until wilted.
3. Whisk eggs and pour over the vegetables.
4. Top with crumbled feta and season with salt and pepper.
5. Bake until set.

Servings: 1

Nutritional Value: Calories: 290, Calcium: 180 mg

Vitamin D: 60 IU

Cooking Time: 20 minutes

7. Lentil and Vegetable Stuffed Peppers

Ingredients:

- Bell peppers, halved and cleaned
- Cooked lentils
- Mixed vegetables (carrots, zucchini, tomatoes)
- Tomato sauce
- Italian seasoning, salt, and pepper to taste

Instructions:

1. Mix cooked lentils, mixed vegetables, tomato sauce, and seasoning.
2. Stuff bell peppers with the mixture.
3. Bake until peppers are tender.

Servings: 1

Nutritional Value:

- Calories: 330
- Calcium: 140 mg
- Vitamin D: 70 IU

Cooking Time: 35 minutes

8. Cauliflower Rice and Chicken Stir-Fry

Ingredients:

- 4 oz cooked chicken breast, sliced
- Cauliflower rice
- Broccoli florets
- Carrots, julienned
- Low-sodium teriyaki sauce
- Olive oil, garlic, ginger, salt, and pepper to taste

Instructions:

1. Sauté chicken, cauliflower rice, broccoli, and carrots in olive oil.
2. Add minced garlic, ginger, and teriyaki sauce.
3. Stir-fry until vegetables are tender.

Servings: 1

Nutritional Value:

- Calories: 380
- Calcium: 160 mg
- Vitamin D: 80 IU

Cooking Time: 20 minutes

9. Cabbage and Lentil Soup

Ingredients:

- Green cabbage, shredded
- Cooked lentils
- Low-sodium vegetable broth
- Onion, garlic, thyme, salt, and pepper to taste

Instructions:

1. Combine shredded cabbage, cooked lentils, and vegetable broth in a pot.
2. Sauté onions and garlic, then add to the soup.
3. Season with thyme, salt, and pepper.
4. Simmer until cabbage is tender.

Servings: 1

Nutritional Value:

- Calories: 290
- Calcium: 140 mg
- Vitamin D: 60 IU

Cooking Time: 30 minutes

10. Turkey and Sweet Potato Skillet

Ingredients:

- Ground turkey
- Sweet potatoes, diced
- Bell peppers, sliced
- Onion, diced
- Olive oil, garlic, paprika, cumin, salt, and pepper to taste

Instructions:

1. Cook ground turkey in olive oil until browned.
2. Add diced sweet potatoes, bell peppers, and onions.
3. Season with minced garlic, paprika, cumin, salt, and pepper.
4. Sauté until sweet potatoes are cooked.

Servings: 1   **Cooking Time:** 25 minutes

Nutritional Value:

- Calories: 350
- Calcium: 120 mg
- Vitamin D: 70 IU

11. Quinoa and Broccoli Bowl with Tofu

Ingredients:

- Cooked quinoa
- Broccoli florets
- Firm tofu, cubed and baked
- Soy sauce
- Sesame oil, garlic, ginger, salt, and pepper to taste

Instructions:

1. Sauté broccoli in sesame oil until tender.
2. Add baked tofu, cooked quinoa, soy sauce, minced garlic, and ginger.
3. Stir-fry until heated through.

Servings: 1

Nutritional Value:

- Calories: 370
- Calcium: 180 mg
- Vitamin D: 90 IU

Cooking Time: 20 minutes

12. Miso-Glazed Cod with Bok Choy

Ingredients:

- Cod fillet
- Bok choy, chopped
- Miso paste
- Low-sodium soy sauce
- Sesame oil, garlic, ginger, salt, and pepper to taste

Instructions:

1. Mix miso paste, soy sauce, minced garlic, and ginger.
2. Brush cod with the miso mixture and bake until cooked.
3. Sauté bok choy in sesame oil.
4. Serve cod over sautéed bok choy.

Servings: 1

Nutritional Value:

- Calories: 320
- Calcium: 160 mg
- Vitamin D: 100 IU

Cooking Time: 20 minutes

13. Chickpea and Spinach Curry

Ingredients:

- Canned chickpeas, rinsed
- Fresh spinach leaves
- Coconut milk
- Curry powder, turmeric, garlic, salt, and pepper to taste

Instructions:

1. Combine chickpeas, spinach, coconut milk, and spices in a pot.
2. Simmer until spinach is wilted and chickpeas are heated through.

Servings: 1

Nutritional Value:

- Calories: 360
- Calcium: 120 mg
- Vitamin D: 70 IU

Cooking Time: 15 minutes

14. Stuffed Acorn Squash with Quinoa

Ingredients:

- Acorn squash, halved and cleaned
- Cooked quinoa
- Diced apples
- Pecans, chopped
- Maple syrup
- Cinnamon, nutmeg, salt, and pepper to taste

Instructions:

1. Mix cooked quinoa, diced apples, chopped pecans, maple syrup, and spices.
2. Stuff acorn squash with the mixture.
3. Bake until squash is tender.

Servings: 1

Nutritional Value:

- Calories: 380
- Calcium: 180 mg
- Vitamin D: 80 IU

Cooking Time: 35 minutes

15. Grilled Portobello Mushrooms with Quinoa

Ingredients:

- Portobello mushrooms, cleaned
- Quinoa, cooked
- Cherry tomatoes, sliced
- Fresh basil leaves
- Balsamic glaze
- Olive oil, garlic, salt, and pepper to taste

Instructions:

1. Grill portobello mushrooms until tender.
2. Mix cooked quinoa, sliced cherry tomatoes, fresh basil, olive oil, minced garlic, and season with salt and pepper.
3. Serve grilled portobellos over quinoa mixture.
4. Drizzle with balsamic glaze.

Servings: 1

Nutritional Value: Calories: 350, Calcium: 150 mg, Vitamin D: 70 IU

Cooking Time: 20 minutes

Snack and dessert Recipes:

1. Greek Yogurt Parfait with Berries

Ingredients:

- 1 cup Greek yogurt
- Mixed berries (blueberries, strawberries)
- Almonds, chopped
- Honey

Instructions:

1. Layer Greek yogurt, mixed berries, and chopped almonds in a glass.
2. Drizzle with honey.

Servings: 1

Nutritional Value:

- Calories: 250
- Calcium: 300 mg
- Vitamin D: 80 IU

2. Cottage Cheese and Pineapple Bowls

Ingredients:

- 1/2 cup low-fat cottage cheese
- Fresh pineapple chunks
- Mint leaves

Instructions:

1. Combine cottage cheese and pineapple in a bowl.
2. Garnish with fresh mint leaves.

Servings: 1

Nutritional Value:

- Calories: 180
- Calcium: 200 mg
- Vitamin D: 60 IU

Ingredients:

- Banana, sliced
- Almond butter
- Almonds, crushed

Instructions:

1. Spread almond butter on banana slices.
2. Sprinkle crushed almonds on top.

Servings: 1

Nutritional Value:

- Calories: 200
- Calcium: 120 mg
- Vitamin D: 40 IU

Ingredients:

- 2 tablespoons chia seeds
- 1/2 cup almond milk
- Kiwi, sliced

Instructions:

1. Mix chia seeds and almond milk in a bowl.
2. Refrigerate until it forms a pudding-like consistency.
3. Top with sliced kiwi.

Servings: 1

Nutritional Value:

- Calories: 180
- Calcium: 160 mg
- Vitamin D: 70 IU

Preparation Time: 2 hours (plus chilling time)

5. Dark Chocolate-Dipped Strawberries

Ingredients:

- Fresh strawberries
- Dark chocolate, melted
- Pistachios, chopped

Instructions:

1. Dip strawberries in melted dark chocolate.
2. Sprinkle chopped pistachios on top.

Servings: 1

Nutritional Value:

- Calories: 150
- Calcium: 80 mg
- Vitamin D: 30 IU

Cooking Time: 10 minutes (plus cooling time)

Ingredients:

- Apple, sliced
- Walnuts, chopped
- Raisins
- Cinnamon

Instructions:

1. Combine sliced apples, chopped walnuts, and raisins in a bowl.
2. Sprinkle with cinnamon.

Servings: 1

Nutritional Value:

- Calories: 200
- Calcium: 120 mg
- Vitamin D: 40 IU

Ingredients:

- Avocado, diced
- Tomato, diced
- Red onion, finely chopped
- Cilantro, chopped
- Lime juice, salt, and pepper to taste

Instructions:

1. Mix diced avocado, tomato, red onion, and cilantro in a bowl.
2. Drizzle with lime juice and season with salt and pepper.
3. Serve with whole-grain crackers.

Servings: 1

Nutritional Value:

- Calories: 220
- Calcium: 80 mg
- Vitamin D: 60 IU

8. Coconut Yogurt and Mango Parfait

Ingredients:

- 1 cup coconut yogurt
- Fresh mango chunks
- Granola

Instructions:

1. Layer coconut yogurt, mango chunks, and granola in a glass.

Servings: 1

Nutritional Value:

- Calories: 280
- Calcium: 250 mg
- Vitamin D: 70 IU

9. Pumpkin Spice Energy Bites

Ingredients:

- 1 cup rolled oats
- Pumpkin puree
- Almond butter
- Pumpkin spice
- Chia seeds

Instructions:

1. Mix rolled oats, pumpkin puree, almond butter, pumpkin spice, and chia seeds.
2. Form into small energy bites.

Servings: 1

Nutritional Value:

- Calories: 180
- Calcium: 120 mg
- Vitamin D: 40 IU

Preparation Time: 15 minutes (plus chilling time)

10. Mango Sorbet

Ingredients:

- Frozen mango chunks
- Coconut water
- Fresh mint leaves

Instructions:

1. Blend frozen mango chunks with coconut water until smooth.
2. Garnish with fresh mint leaves.

Servings: 1

Nutritional Value:

- Calories: 120
- Calcium: 40 mg
- Vitamin D: 50 IU

Preparation Time: 5 minutes

11. Cucumber and Hummus Rolls

Ingredients:

- Cucumber, thinly sliced
- Hummus
- Cherry tomatoes, sliced

Instructions:

1. Spread hummus on cucumber slices.
2. Place a slice of cherry tomato on each and roll up.

Servings: 1

Nutritional Value:

- Calories: 130
- Calcium: 60 mg
- Vitamin D: 30 IU

12. Berry and Almond Smoothie Bowl

Ingredients:

- Mixed berries (strawberries, blueberries, raspberries)
- Almond milk
- Almond butter
- Granola

Instructions:

1. Blend mixed berries, almond milk, and almond butter until smooth.
2. Pour into a bowl and top with granola.

Servings: 1

Nutritional Value:

- Calories: 230
- Calcium: 120 mg
- Vitamin D: 60 IU

Preparation Time: 10 minutes

13. Peach and Mint Salsa

Ingredients:

- Fresh peaches, diced
- Red bell pepper, diced
- Red onion, finely chopped
- Fresh mint leaves, chopped
- Lime juice, salt, and pepper to taste

Instructions:

1. Mix diced peaches, bell pepper, red onion, and mint in a bowl.
2. Drizzle with lime juice and season with salt and pepper.
3. Serve with whole-grain pita chips.

Servings: 1

Nutritional Value:

- Calories: 180
- Calcium: 60 mg
- Vitamin D: 50 IU

14. Cherry Almond Frozen Yogurt Popsicles

Ingredients:

- Greek yogurt
- Cherries, pitted and halved
- Almonds, chopped

Instructions:

1. Mix Greek yogurt, cherry halves, and chopped almonds.
2. Pour into popsicle molds and freeze.

Servings: 1

Nutritional Value:

- Calories: 160
- Calcium: 100 mg
- Vitamin D: 30 IU

Preparation Time: 10 minutes (plus freezing time)

Ingredients:

- Watermelon, cut into cubes
- Feta cheese, cubed
- Fresh mint leaves

Instructions:

1. Thread watermelon cubes, feta cheese, and mint leaves onto skewers.

Servings: 1

Nutritional Value:

- Calories: 120
- Calcium: 80 mg
- Vitamin D: 40 IU

Enjoy your healthy delicious meal!!!!

CONCLUSION

The "Osteoporosis Diet Cookbook for Seniors" is not just a collection of recipes; it is a holistic guide crafted with care and expertise to empower older individuals on their journey toward better bone health. The carefully curated chapters cover the essential aspects of understanding osteoporosis, identifying risk factors, and embracing a diet rich in calcium and nutrients vital for bone strength.

This cookbook transcends the realm of mere recipes; it becomes a companion for those navigating the challenges of osteoporosis. By delving into the impact of osteoporosis on senior health, uncovering risk factors, and elucidating the roles of calcium, vitamins, and minerals, it equips readers with knowledge to make informed dietary choices.

The diverse recipes presented here, from nutrient-dense plant-based options to smart meal planning for bone health, offer a flavorful journey toward better well-being.

Each recipe is a testament to the idea that eating for bone health can be both delicious and purposeful. From breakfast to dinner, snacks to desserts, the cookbook caters to varied tastes while adhering to the principles of a diet beneficial for osteoporosis management.

Dear reader, adopting this cookbook isn't just about embracing a set of recipes; it's about embracing a lifestyle that champions your bone health. As you savor the delightful flavors of these thoughtfully crafted dishes, envision each bite as a step toward stronger bones and a more resilient you. Nourish not just your body but your spirit, for every meal is an opportunity to invest in your long-term well-being. Let the joy of cooking become the joy of taking charge of your health. Embrace this cookbook, savor the flavors, and relish the journey to stronger, healthier bones— one delicious meal at a time.

Your bones, your vitality, and your future self will thank you.

MEAL PLANNER

DATE:

	BREAKFAST	LUNCH	DINNER	SHOPPING LIST
MON				
TUES				
WED				
THURS				
FRI				
SAT				
SUN				

MEAL PLANNER

DATE:

	BREAKFAST	LUNCH	DINNER	SHOPPING LIST
MON				
TUES				
WED				
THURS				
FRI				
SAT				
SUN				

MEAL PLANNER

DATE:

	BREAKFAST	LUNCH	DINNER	SHOPPING LIST
MON				
TUES				
WED				
THURS				
FRI				
SAT				
SUN				

MEAL PLANNER

DATE:

	BREAKFAST	LUNCH	DINNER	SHOPPING LIST
MON				
TUES				
WED				
THURS				
FRI				
SAT				
SUN				

MEAL PLANNER

DATE:

	BREAKFAST	LUNCH	DINNER	SHOPPING LIST
MON				
TUES				
WED				
THURS				
FRI				
SAT				
SUN				

MEAL PLANNER

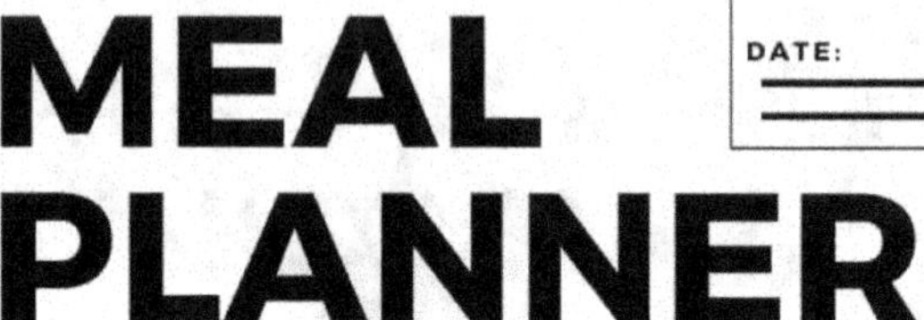

DATE:

	BREAKFAST	LUNCH	DINNER	SHOPPING LIST
MON				
TUES				
WED				
THURS				
FRI				
SAT				
SUN				

MEAL PLANNER

DATE:

	BREAKFAST	LUNCH	DINNER	SHOPPING LIST
MON				
TUES				
WED				
THURS				
FRI				
SAT				
SUN				

MEAL PLANNER

DATE:

	BREAKFAST	LUNCH	DINNER	SHOPPING LIST
MON				
TUES				
WED				
THURS				
FRI				
SAT				
SUN				

MEAL PLANNER

DATE:

	BREAKFAST	LUNCH	DINNER	SHOPPING LIST
MON				
TUES				
WED				
THURS				
FRI				
SAT				
SUN				

MEAL PLANNER

DATE:

	BREAKFAST	LUNCH	DINNER	SHOPPING LIST
MON				
TUES				
WED				
THURS				
FRI				
SAT				
SUN				

MEAL PLANNER

DATE:

	BREAKFAST	LUNCH	DINNER	SHOPPING LIST
MON				
TUES				
WED				
THURS				
FRI				
SAT				
SUN				

MEAL PLANNER

DATE:

	BREAKFAST	LUNCH	DINNER	SHOPPING LIST
MON				
TUES				
WED				
THURS				
FRI				
SAT				
SUN				

MEAL PLANNER

DATE:

	BREAKFAST	LUNCH	DINNER	SHOPPING LIST
MON				
TUES				
WED				
THURS				
FRI				
SAT				
SUN				

MEAL PLANNER

DATE:

	BREAKFAST	LUNCH	DINNER	SHOPPING LIST
MON				
TUES				
WED				
THURS				
FRI				
SAT				
SUN